101 Simple Things You Can Do To Stay on a Diet And Lose Weight!

By Doug Kirkpatrick

Baker Publishing

**Copyright © 1992 Douglas Kirkpatrick
All rights reserved.**

Published by Baker Publishing P.O. Box 8341 Mission Hills, CA 91346. No part of this book may be reproduced or transmitted by any means, electronic or mechanical, including photocopying, without written permission from the publisher, except for brief quotations in articles and reviews.

Notice - This book is intended as a reference only and not as a medical guide for self-treatment. It is not intended as a substitue for medical advice or treatment from your doctor. In addition, you are urged to consult your doctor before dieting or engaging in any exercise program. Neither the publisher nor the author shall be liable to the purchaser or any other person or persons for loss or damage caused or alleged to have been caused directly or indirectly by the use of the information contained in this book.

**ISBN: 0-913193-04-6
Library of Congress: 91-076748**

Printed in the United States of America
987654321

Contents

Preface
The Conspiracy 5
Many Diets, Much Confusion 7
Why Diets Fail 9
Diet Traps to Avoid 13
The Real Secret of Losing Weight 16
The Best Diet in the World 17
How to Stay on Any Diet 19
How to Eliminate Poor Eating Habits ... 25
101 Simple Things You Can Do:
    The Basics 29
    At Home 65
    Exercise 85
    Shopping For Food 95
    When Dining Out 112
    At Parties, Receptions, Etc. 107
    At The Office 121
    Final Tip 127
Do a Friend a Favor 128

Preface

Are you frustrated because you are unable to lose weight and keep it off? Do you slip back into old eating habits after dieting only to regain all the weight you have lost and sometimes even more?

For almost two decades this was the trap I found myself in. Time and time again, I would become motivated, lose weight, and then regain what I had lost. After much frustraton, I started asking others how they were able to lose weight and keep it off. From their success stories, I learned many practical ideas. But above all, I discovered I also had to change *why* I ate. This book is a collection of those ideas and shows you how to make the changes necessary to lose weight once and for all.

The Conspiracy

Whether you know it or not, there is a plan to sabotage your diet. Its conspirators include your family and friends, the advertising industry, multinational corporations, as well as yourself. Many times family and friends unknowingly undermine your diet. They show their love and affection with mass quantities of food and drink at parties, gatherings, and during the holidays.

Too often these occasions are remembered by what was served and how much was consumed. Unfortunately, this type of caring and hospitality has linked and associated overeating to the joys we get from being with our families and friends. Bad eating habits are reinforced without us knowing what's really going on.

But let's be honest. When it comes to dieting, we are our own worst enemies. We contribute to our own downfall from the meanings and associations we have placed on food. In our abundant society consuming food has become much more than something we do just to survive. Much too often we eat to feed and satisfy our emotions. Without even knowing it, we form and reward eating habits that conflict with our desire to be thin.

But failure to stay on a diet is not entirely your fault or that of well-meaning family and friends. Food advertisers are also to blame. They condition us to eat more by spending millions. Remember the Burger King commercial that kept asking *"Aren't you hungry?"* Food and beverage advertisers want us to associate the good times in life with consuming their products! Pay close attention to their commericals and you'll see what I mean.

Many Diets – Much Confusion

To counter this avalanche of advertising pressure, we spend billions of dollars every year on diet doctors, pills, health spas, diet books, subliminal audio tapes, weight loss clinics, cosmetic surgery, and even hypnotists. We do this to take off what others have encouraged us to put on. It just doesn't seem fair does it?

Then, when you have finally said to yourself "**I've had it!**" and determined to do something about all those extra pounds, there are so many different diets. And don't forget about the countless celebrities promoting their diet books, weight loss programs, and exercise videos.

Unfortunately, many claim that their diet program is the simplest, the best, the fastest, or the healthiest. In all fairness, some diets being promoted are good, others really don't help you lose weight, while a few can actually be dangerous to your health.

But how do you know whose claims to believe? And which diet will help you achieve your desired weight? Before that secret is revealed, let's first look at why diets fail.

Why Diets Fail

Here are the six basic reasons why diets fail:

1) *Procrastination* - First, you must get started. Many people find that this is the most difficult part of dieting. They simply keep making excuses why they cannot or should not start losing weight until after some event takes place. Too often these excuses involve the dinner party next weekend, a special meal you've been looking forward to, or tonight's trip to the ice cream store. Procrastination is the first major obstacle to overcome in dieting. Just take action and begin your diet now.

2) *Lack of Desire and Motivation* - It takes effort to maintain desire and motivation once you have decided to take action and lose weight. It's just too easy to

lose interest or get side tracked in the middle of your diet. This happens frequently when you don't see immediate results. The key is to keep your focus and concentrate on what you want over the long term. Don't give in to the short term pleasure of a candy bar or banana split over the long range benefits of better health and an improved self image. Why not just put off having those treats until after you have achieved your goal? (However, reward yourself in moderation and it's better to use something other than food.)

3) *Poor Eating Habits* **-** Consuming the wrong foods, eating too much, eating to satisfy feelings, eating to overcome emotions, and eating as a reaction to stress are examples of poor, if not self-destructive, eating habits. If these habits are not changed, they will always override the desire and willpower needed to reach your dieting goals. It's just too easy to cheat without thinking about what you are doing. The key to losing weight and keeping it off is to eliminate your poor eating habits.

4) *Not Being Honest with Yourself* - Many unsuccessful dieters constantly fool themselves. They think they are actually eating less than they really are. The problem is that they conveniently forget about that extra nibble or treat they have consumed. Also, they don't feel that serving sizes make a difference as long as a particular food is on their diet. Many of these dieters actually eat more than before they went on their so-called "diet" and gain additional pounds. Dishonest dieters wonder why diets just don't work for them. If you are sincere about losing weight, it's not hard to be honest with yourself about your eating habits.

5) *Poor Planning* - Diets fail because of unstructured eating patterns caused by poor planning. Unstructured eating means consuming meals and snacks that are not part your diet plan. Sometimes you simply have not considered the right foods and quantities you must eat to lose weight. A diet specialist or doctor can help you here. In addition, many times it is difficult to maintain structure when you are away from home, at parties, and at restaurants.

6) *Belief in Diet Myths* – Finally, many unsuccessful dieters look for the short cut or an instant solution for losing weight. They are easily influenced by anyone who tells them what they want to hear. Because some diet myths are repeated so often, many people accept them without question. These myths trap would-be dieters into to unrealistic expectations for losing weight.

Diet Traps to Avoid

There are many dieting myths about rapid weight loss methods. Unfortunately, many people have put their faith into one or more of these dieting techniques only to be disappointed. These myths trap you into a short term solution while setting you up for the long term frustration of never reaching or maintaining your ideal weight.

Fad Diet Trap - After the frustration of losing and regaining weight, it's very easy to be sold on any new diet that promises to be fast and easy. The trap is that many fad diets promise quick weight loss but never deal with permanent weight loss. It's a good bet that any weight lost on one of these diets will be regained. Sadly, some fad diets have even been proven to be dangerous to your health because they don't provide proper nutrition. It is better to stay with a diet that has already been proven to work safely for others and not risk your health. And besides, how many fad diets can you remember that have withstood the test of time?

Calories Don't Count Trap - Some diets want you to believe that you don't need to watch how much you eat or even count calories as long as you only eat certain foods. The truth is that calories do count. In fact, calories are the only thing that counts. Once consumed, a calorie is either used by the body or stored as fat. Bottom line: if you eat and don't use the calories, you wear them.

Crash Diets and Fasting Traps - These methods for losing weight put a tremendous strain on your body and its digestive system. And you will not get essential vitamins, minerals, and other nutrients without taking supplements. Simply put, why would you want to risk your health when there are better ways to adjust your eating habits for permanent weight loss? In addition, crash diets and fasting lead you into the next trap of yo-yo dieting.

Yo-Yo Dieting Trap - This trap is the endless cycle of gaining weight by overeating and then taking it off by extreme dieting. At best, this behavior promotes and reinforces the poor eating habits you must change for permanent weight loss. At worst, it can lead to eating disorders such as binging and purging. And like fasting and crash dieting, large and rapid changes in your weight can put a tremendous strain on your body.

The Real Secret of Losing Weight

How does anyone lose weight? Simple. So simple in fact, many people are convinced that it just has to be more difficult.

Here's the secret - In order to lose weight all you have to do is:

1) Eat less than is necessary to maintain your current weight.

or

2) Burn more calories through activity and exercise while maintaining the same food intake.

It's that simple. The hard part is taking action and staying with it until you succeed.

The Best Diet in the World

Taking into consideration everything discussed so far, and without further ado, here is the answer you have been waiting for ...

Question -
 What is the best diet in the world?

Answer -
 The one you can and will stay with!

Diets don't work if you are not committed. All long term results depend on commitment and your ability to change eating habits. Also, a diet plan will only do certain things for you. It will tell you what and how much to eat while helping to plan meals. However, a diet won't give you the reinforcement necessary to stay with it. This is where that space between your ears becomes so important. You must ultimately change your eating habits and patterns to lose weight permanently. Remember, no diet book or doctor can do that for you.

Important – It's always a good idea to have your doctor review, approve, and supervise your diet. Many times just cutting back on snacking and your total food intake is enough to lose the weight. But if you have a great deal of weight to lose, you should consult your doctor or a weight loss specialist before doing something that could affect your health.

How to Stay on Any Diet

The secret of losing weight depends on your ability to stay with your diet plan until you succeed. Here are the ten keys:

Desire - Desire comes from a combination of two sources. The first is from the rational and well thought out reasons why you want or need to lose weight. Reasons are definitely a good start, but too often results don't come from logical or rational thoughts alone.

This brings us to the second and most important component of desire. Lasting desire comes from internalizing the reasons *why* you want to lose weight. Reasons combined with feelings and emotions push you into taking action. Sometimes this involves moving away from the feelings our present condition gives us. Other times this involves the positive feelings we get from thinking about what reaching our goal would mean. The stronger our feelings, the stronger our desire. Whether we want to move towards a positive result or away from our current condition, desire is where every successful diet starts. If you don't have the desire, any diet will fail and you will go back to old eating habits quickly.

Belief - Believe that you can lose weight and you will lose weight. Belief will carry you in the beginning and through difficult times. Without belief you will only make half-hearted attempts to shed those extra pounds. It's too easy to become discouraged, make an excuse, and then give up. Remember, whether you think you can do something or you think you can't, **you're right!**

Willpower - Willpower starts with your desire. It is your determination to stay the course and is important when starting a new diet. Willpower is really not hard to establish once you understand why you overeat. Give yourself enough good reasons and you can do anything. The good news is that once your eating habits start to change, willpower becomes less important in maintaining your diet.

Structure - The best way to maintain a diet is by giving it structure. For example, try consuming your meals at the same times and in the same places according to a pre-planned menu. Structure helps establish new eating habits and patterns. Unfortunately, maintaining diet structure can be difficult especially for those who travel frequently. The key is to set up a routine for eating and to stay with it no matter where you are.

Constant Reminders - Reminders keep your mind focused and help you concentrate on what you are trying to accomplish. When you set yourself up to be reminded regularly as to why you want to lose weight, you will find it easier to maintain desire and willpower. They can be as simple as an index card with your desired weight and the benefits you will get from reaching it. Constant reminders help you stay with your diet and reach your goal.

Physical Barriers - Another method that has helped many people stay on their diet is to place physical barriers between them and food. These barriers can be as simple as storing food where it is inconvenient to get to or as complex as locking food up and giving someone else the key. Barriers are not a permanent solution to staying on a diet, but they are helpful in building momentum in your weight loss program.

Psychological Deterrents - These are similar to constant reminders but tend to emphasize the negative side of not staying on your diet. A good example is placing a recent picture of yourself on the refrigerator. The purpose is to show you what you want to to change about yourself just as you reach for a snack.

Visualize Benefits - It is much easier to maintain your desire and motivation for dieting by seeing and experiencing the benefits in advance. First, picture in your mind's eye exactly what you will look like after reaching your goal. Then put this new image of yourself into situations that previously made you uncomfortable because of your weight. Finally, carry this mental image with you and continue to enjoying the positive feeling it gives you.

Eliminate Poor Eating Habits - Most people think that it's next to impossible to eliminate a habit. This is especially true for an eating habit that gives them pleasure or is a substitute for something missing in their lives. Unfortunately, many of us have associated and linked feelings and emotions with food. For example, some people get feelings of comfort by eating. Others get positive feelings and a sense of reward from food. The point is that everybody has their own reasons why they overeat. The first step in eliminating a habit is to understand *why* you do what you do. Also, a habit is not hard to change or eliminate once you know how. Unfortunately, most people don't know where to start or what to do.

Have Patience - Give your diet plan a chance to work and don't become discouraged. Eating habits can be changed as you will soon see.

How to Eliminate Poor Eating Habits

If you have stayed with me, you have seen that you must change your eating habits and patterns to stay on a diet, lose weight, and to ultimately keep it off. Here are the five steps necessary in eliminating poor eating habits:

1) Identify and understand exactly what eating habit you need to eliminate. For example; do you eat for immediate gratification and pleasure, or to satisfy a need that you feel can only be done through eating? Do you eat to change your mood or state of mind such as boredom or loneliness? Do you eat as a reaction to stress or pressure? Do you eat because of habits learned and reinforced in childhood such as being rewarded with something to eat or drink for good behavior?

2) Convince yourself that it is absolutely necessary that you change your behavior. Wanting to change is not enough. Keep focused on the benefits and rewards for changing and the penalties or costs for not doing so. The idea is to get enough leverage on yourself to make the change.

3) Determine exactly what stimulus triggers the undesirable eating behavior. Many times there are multiple triggers that result in overeating. The trick is finding out which ones affect your behavior. Just becoming aware of these triggers is 90% of the battle. Stop yourself just before eating something you had not planned on and isolate exactly what you were feeling, doing, and thinking about.

4) Take action immediately the next time one of these stimuli or triggers occur. The purpose is to interrupt your state of mind and pattern of behavior. You must turn off your automatic pilot and take control. One of the easiest and fastest ways to change your state is through your physiology or body movement. For example; try exercising, deep breathing, or doing something physical that redirects your focus away from stuffing food into your mouth. Do this enough times and the trigger no longer results in the automatic reaction of eating.

5) Keep at it. Persist in eliminating your poor eating habits. It may take three to four weeks to overcome some habits that have been practiced and reinforced over a lifetime. The point is to keep trying and not give up.

Once desirable eating patterns are established, they become second nature or what is commonly referred to as a *good habit*. Failing to understand this key point, you will never get out of the cycle that "diets are forever".

Now, get ready for the 101 simple things you can do to stay on a diet and lose weight!

The Basics ...

<u>1</u>

Start your diet right now. I mean right now! Not tonight at dinner, not next week or after the party on Saturday, right now. If you are serious and committed, it is easy to begin this very minute.

2

Choose a diet, with the help of your doctor, that has been proven over time to be both safe and effective for losing weight. There is really no valid reason to experiment with a new or fad diet when you know of a diet that has worked for others.

3

Find someone who has been successful in losing weight and keeping it off. Then ask that person how he or she lost the weight and what problems were encountered. When dieting, it is easier and faster to learn from someone else by modeling their actions.

4

Don't take drugs or diet pills to depress your appetite. It's better to teach your brain to control how and when to eat rather than to rely on drugs for losing weight. This method is much safer too.

5

Set realistic goals and timetables for losing weight. Most importantly, your weight loss goals and timetables should not jeopardize your health by trying to lose weight too quickly. And second, your goals should be just out of reach and not out of sight. You don't want to become discouraged by just missing or never reaching your objectives.

6

Have a plan for what, when, where, why, and how much you will be eating. Many times just cutting out snacks or reducing the size of food servings is enough to lose the weight. If you need help in choosing the right foods, there are many good diets available in book stores and libraries. (But also remember to consult your doctor.) Then take action and just do it.

7

Log everything you eat to determine exactly what and how much you consume. Also write down when and where you consume food and the mood you are in at the time. This is the fastest way to find out why you overeat and to identify poor eating habits. I know that you are saying to yourself, "Do I really have to do this?" Of course you don't, but why not try it if you have had trouble staying on previous diets? You will probably be surprised to find out how much your really eat.

8

Keep a daily log of your weight to check your progress. However, it's important not to get discouraged if your weight goes up occasionally. Be concerned only with total weekly losses instead of daily fluctuations.

<u>9</u>

Link and associate the pain of not dieting to all things you have missed out on while being overweight. These include outdoor activities, social functions, and contact with others.

10

In your mind, link and associate the pleasure of being successful in accomplishing your goal of losing weight.

11

Put a rubber band on your wrist. Gently snap this "bio feedback" device every time you cheat or even consider cheating on your diet. The purpose is to link a small punishment or pain to the eating habit you want to eliminate.

<u>12</u>

Make a pact with someone else who wants to lose weight. Conduct weekly weigh-ins with the loser doing something for the winner. However, don't make the prize a meal or some other food item. It is important to break the association of winning with eating.

13

Start a support group of friends or co-workers to discuss problems of losing weight and staying on diets. This is one reason why Weight Watchers® and some of the other commercial dieting programs are so successful.

14

Make a bet with a friend or relative that you can lose a given amount of weight by a certain date. (Again, don't make the prize food.) Be sure to make the amount of weight something you can realistically take off without hurting yourself. Then remember to live up to your responsibility if you lose the wager.

<u>15</u>

Learn and then practice the visualization technique of picturing yourself at your ideal weight walking on the beach, at the pool, or being with someone you are attracted to.

16

Refrain from drinking alcohol while on your diet. In addition to saving calories, alcohol can lower your willpower and resistance to cheating. This is especially important at parties where a lot of unstructured eating will be done.

17

Make positive statements out loud about your intentions and goals for losing weight. Do this when you get up in the morning and just before going to bed. The purpose is to implant desire and convince your subconscious that you can achieve your goal of staying on a diet and losing weight. To some this may sound silly but it really does work. It's all in your attitude.

<u>18</u>

Look at yourself naked in the mirror. (Sometimes the shock alone is equal to a week of positive statements!)

19

Learn to recognize if and when you use food to change your mood or state. Then learn other ways to change your state of mind. You can do this by breathing deeply, exercising, and by using visual or auditory stimuli to break your behavior patterns.

20

Learn to recognize if and when you reward yourself with food. The purpose is to identify and change the reward to something other than food.

<u>21</u>

Buy a new suit or other piece of clothing in the size for your ideal weight. Then hang it where you will see it every day. This gives you additional motivation to get down to the weight where you can wear it comfortably.

22

Make and carry index cards with reasons why you want and need to lose weight with the consequences for not succeeding. Read them each morning, noon, and night. Also refer to them just before eating or snacking.

23

Make a written contract with yourself. It should include a reward for reaching your dieting goal and a penalty for not achieving it. The reward could be a vacation, a new wardrobe, or something that will show off the new and improved you. Review this contract daily.

24

Buy a good quality scale that is accurate to within one quarter pound. An inaccurate scale can give positive feedback when it is not deserved and negative feedback when it is.

25

Don't take cooking or cake decorating classes when trying to lose weight. It's just too tempting to eat your homework. Besides, who needs Julia Child as a role model anyway? (Just kidding Julia.)

26

Don't skip meals. Eat smaller portions instead. This is healthier and prevents long periods of feeling hungry.

27

Drink at least three to four extra glasses of water per day. Drink a glass of water instead of snacking. Not only does the water flush out your system while putting something into your stomach, just think of the exercise you'll get by running to the rest-room.

28

Eliminate all fried foods while on your diet. Frying can double the calories in a food. Instead; bake, steam, microwave, or broil your foods to reduce both calories and fat.

29

Notice how fast you eat in relation to others dining with you. You may have a tendency to overeat as you wait for others to finish. One way to counter this is to get up and take your plate and utensils away from the table or have them removed at a restaurant.

30

Don't change your eating patterns or habits on weekends. Many people make the mistake of using food to celebrate when they are able to make it through another week.

31

Go "cold turkey" on desserts while dieting. It is surprising, but after a few days you won't miss them. If you must have something, substitute low calorie Jell-O® or fruit. Don't eat ice cream, cakes, or other high calorie treats.

<u>32</u>

Unless the diet you are using says it is alright to do so, don't substitute foods or improvise on your own.

33

Dress in tight fitting clothing or wear a tight belt while on a diet. This maybe uncomfortable but it will be a constant reminder not to snack between meals or to overeat.

34

Don't give up on your diet too soon. Give it a chance to work. But if the diet you have chosen is difficult to stay on or does not produce results, by all means don't be afraid to try a different one.

35

Don't automatically give up if you forget once in a while and eat something not on your diet. Small upward fluctuations in your weight should not be a reason for quitting. Remember, you are in it for the long run and the long term benefits. Don't give yourself any excuses, either consciously or subconsciously, for quitting your diet.

<u>36</u>

Carry this book with you for motivation and as a reminder not to lose sight of your goal. In addition, you will burn approximately five calories by lugging it around for a month.

At Home ...

37

Start by getting rid of all unnecessary foods and their containers. This includes plates, trays, candy dishes, and food hidden around the house in case of "an emergency". Also clean out the refrigerator, freezer, and pantry. Get rid of cookies, cakes, candies, potato chips, and all other fattening snacks.

38

Don't keep junk foods or desserts in your home. They are just too tempting to pass up. Remember, out of sight, out of mind.

39

Store all foods out of sight in a pantry or cupboard. Many times just the sight of food triggers some people to start snacking. (Remember the story of Ivan Pavlov's experiment of ringing bells to make dogs salivate?)

40

Plan your meals a week in advance. This gives your diet structure. Planning also helps with shopping by knowing what and how much to buy.

41

Plan and eat meals at specific times. Try to maintain a schedule for eating while on your diet. You want to establish new patterns of behavior and reset your internal "meal clock".

<u>42</u>

Wear a surgical, medical, or dust mask while preparing meals. This sounds silly but makes it extremely hard to nibble or snack before it is time to sit down and eat.

43

Cook and freeze your meals ahead of time. By doing this, you won't have the time or opportunity to snack while preparing them. In addition, many diet programs such as Nutri/System® and Jenny Craig™ use prepared meals to control what and how much to eat. Why not save money by doing it yourself?

<u>44</u>

Eat only at the kitchen or dining room table. This works to limit how much you eat by restricting where you eat it. And, besides, just think of how much you'll save on carpet cleaning.

<u>45</u>

Don't have self-serve, buffet, or "family style" meals at home. Always prepare plates in the kitchen or away from the dinner table. It's just too easy to take more food than you really need. This also makes second helpings more difficult to get.

46

Have your meals served on small plates. The idea is to take less food and to fool your eyes and stomach.

47

Leave the food serving plates in the kitchen and not on the dinner table. Don't make second helpings easy to get. It's even better to put leftovers immediately into the refrigerator before sitting down to eat.

<u>48</u>

Eat a sensible breakfast when dieting. Do not skip this meal trying to save extra calories. It is better to put something in your stomach to give you energy, to keep you from feeling hungry, and to prevent you from overeating at lunch.

49

Eat slowly using small bites and put your fork down after every bite. The purpose is to eat less in a given time. This may be difficult at first because many overweight people tend to eat rapidly. Give this a try, it does work.

50

Store prepared foods and leftovers in containers that you cannot see into. Again, the idea is out of sight, out of mind.

51

Don't clean your plate or feel that you must eat absolutely everything. Many times the urge to finish everything, even when you are full, is a bad habit that was formed when growing up. Remember the story about the starving kids in China your parents told to get you to clean your plate. I hope you don't use it on your kids!

52

Freeze leftovers or throw them out immediately so you won't be tempted to finish them. It's bad form to eat the leftovers and then rationalize that you needed to save space in the refrigerator.

53

Put a scale in front of your refrigerator as a deterrent and friendly reminder that you will be weighing yourself regularly to check your diet progress.

54

Then, put a picture of yourself on the refrigerator. This creates a strong link between food and what you want to change about yourself.

55

Don't eat while reading. If you need something to do with your hands while reading, hold on to a string of beads or squeeze a tennis ball. If you need an additional distraction while reading, turn on the TV or the radio instead of snacking.

<u>56</u>

Don't eat after 8 pm and don't go to bed on a full stomach.

<u>57</u>

In addition, don't eat in bed. If tired or bored, don't use food to change your mood or help you sleep. Eating in bed can become a habit very quickly.

58

Don't eat while watching television. Try knitting, sewing, or working on some other craft if you need something to occupy your hands. Just don't use food.

Exercise ...

<u>59</u>

It is better to start on a supervised exercise program than to take drugs or diet pills to speed up the weight loss process. Besides increasing the number of calories burned, exercise will help tone your body as a bonus. (Always consult your doctor before starting an exercise program.)

60

Start a regular exercise program to relieve stress. Many people eat more and snack between meals as a reaction to stress or as a means to cope with it. In addition, some authorities claim exercise can actually reduce your appetite.

61

Take a 30 minute walk daily. Do this early in the morning, before work, at lunch, or in the evening. By doing this, you will burn approximately 1200 to 1700 extra calories per week which is the equivalent of one to two pounds per month.

<u>62</u>

Make a commitment to stay with your exercise program just like the commitment you're making to stay on your diet.

63

Remember, your purpose in exercising is not to wear yourself out. It is more important do a little exercise every day rather than over-doing it only one day a week.

64

Make exercising a family affair. Start by taking walks with your spouse and kids. It is a great way to get some exercise while spending time with your family.

65

Take up a sport with someone else wanting to lose weight. Good examples are tennis and racketball. You will have someone to support your diet goals while creating some friendly competition.

66

Make exercise fun and interesting. Go on nature walks to learn more about our environment or take bicycle trips in the countryside.

<u>67</u>

Do both strength and aerobic exercises. According to some training experts, this combination reduces body fat faster than one type of exercise alone. (Again, consult your doctor before hand.)

<u>68</u>

Find an exercise that fits your personality. If you enjoy being by yourself, try walking, swimming, or bicycling. If you like to be sociable, try a team sport like basketball, softball, or ice hockey.

Shopping For Food ...

<u>69</u>

Go shopping for food only when you need to replenish your pantry. Frequent and unplanned shopping trips promote buying the wrong foods and other fattening impulse items.

<u>70</u>

Use a shopping list which includes how much of the foods you need. Otherwise, the tendency is to buy more food than necessary and to purchase items not on your diet.

71

Don't shop when you're hungry. Otherwise, you will usually buy more food than you need and will purchase snacks and other items not on your diet.

<u>72</u>

Don't eat while shopping for food. With all those tempting goodies in the market, it's just to easy too fall off your diet.

__73__

Many of us are unaware of just how many calories or grams of fat most of our foods contain. Buy and study books such as the *T-Factor Fat Gram Counter* and the *Vest Pocket Calorie Counter*. They will make you aware of high calorie, high fat foods you should avoid buying.

__74__

Then, read the labels on the foods you buy, especially the prepared foods. This will make you aware of the amount of fat and calories they contain as well as the nutritional values.

<u>75</u>

Switch to low calorie versions of the same foods you currently buy. Try tuna packed in water instead of oil, skim or 1% low fat milk instead of whole milk, non fat yogurt instead of low fat, canned fruit packed in its own juices instead of heavy syrup.

76

Shop for the leanest cuts of meat your can find. Then purchase the cuts graded as "select" rather than "choice" or "prime" which contain more fat and calories. As for poultry, buy chicken and turkey breasts rather than the dark meat cuts. Don't buy self-basting turkeys which use added fats and oils to give you that golden brown skin color. Also avoid duck and goose. Finally, reduce the size of meat servings and include more vegetables and other low calorie side dishes.

77

Don't fall into the "light" or "lite" food trap. A food designated as "light" or "lite" only has to have 33% less calories than the original. Almost no light food is really low in calories with one exception. I've been told there is a "light" water imported from South America. (Light water? *You've got to be kidding!*) One food manufacturer was asked about why its light version of a product had the same amount of calories as the original. The company responded by stating that the "lite" referred to the texture. (Yeah, right!) So check the labels and compare. And remember, it is still important to be concerned about exactly how much of a "light" or "lite" food you consume.

__78__

When buying prepared foods that list calories per serving, be sure to check the size of the serving. Is the serving size enough for a real meal? Sometimes food manufacturers will use the serving size trick to claim that the low calorie version of the product has half the calories or fat of the original while forgetting to tell you that the serving size is only one half the size of the original.

79

Check how the manufacturer measures the amount of fat in its product. Is fat measured as a percentage of the total weight of the product or is it measured in total grams of fat? When measured as a percentage, the true fat content can be distorted in the consumer's mind especially when the product contains heavy ingredients like milk.

80

Pay close attention to the labels on mineral or seltzer waters. You may be thinking, "Water doesn't have calories, does it?" However, some bottled waters have added sweeteners and contain calories you normally would not expect.

When Dining Out ...

<u>81</u>

Know basically what you are going to order before entering a restaurant or seeing the menu. Also, make your mind up ahead of time that you don't need or want an appetizer or dessert. The purpose is to reinforce the idea that you are going to order something that fits into your diet.

82

Don't go to all you can eat restaurants or order the buffet. It's too easy to fill your plate and consume more than you should.

83

Don't sit in the bar when waiting to be seated at a restaurant. It is too easy to eat bar snacks while ordering appetizers and an extra round of drinks that you really don't need.

84

Order a la carte rather than having a complete meal with soup, salad, and dessert. This way you are served just what you need to stay on your diet. (Also saves money too!)

85

When eating out, don't be afraid to ask for meals prepared specifically with your diet in mind. Request to have your food broiled or baked instead of fried. Also ask if the restaurant offers low calorie meals not listed on the menu.

86

Don't eat bread or rolls, especially with butter, while waiting to be served. You will be full before your meal arrives and end up stuffing yourself trying to finish the main course. Simply ask the waiter to take them away so you won't be tempted.

<u>87</u>

Close your eyes or excuse yourself from the table when the waiter brings the dessert tray. (Remember the conspiracy I told you about on page 5?)

88

Don't feel you must finish your entire meal. Ask for a doggie bag if it's against your nature to waste food.

At Parties, Receptions, Etc. ...

89

Don't go to a party or get-together feeling hungry. Even at a sit down dinner there are usually hor d'oeuvres and other fattening munchies to fill up on before the meal is served. It is better to eat some low calorie fruit or vegetables before arriving.

90

Anticipate that there will be large quantities of food and snacks available at a party. Before arriving, picture in your mind exactly what you will eat and what you will pass up, then stick to it. Don't go into a high risk situation without a plan.

__91__

If you are on a diet that uses prepared meals, don't be afraid to bring them to the party. Most people will understand if you advise your host or hostess when you accept the invitation. Besides, dieting is not a valid reason for missing a party.

92

Don't wait until after a holiday to start your diet. (See Tip #1 on page 29.) By not eating sensibly, you will have even more weight to lose later. There is no reason you can't eat intelligently and still enjoy yourself at a holiday gathering. Also, it's a big mistake to use food or drink as a method to get "into the spirit".

93

Instead of alcohol, drink diet soda or sparkling water at parties and receptions. These drinks give you something to fill your hand with instead of high calorie snacks. Also, drinking alcohol helps you forget about your diet while making it easy to revert to nonstop snacking.

94

When you host a party, send a small "care package" home with your guests made from the leftover goodies. The idea is to get all the extra desserts and fattening munchies out of the house. Remember how your mother used this technique on you? (And you thought she was just trying to be nice.)

At the Office ...

<u>95</u>

Take your lunch to work rather than eating out. It's easier to control exactly what your food intake will be.

96

Don't keep food in your desk. Your goal is to make it as hard as possible to fall off your diet plan.

97

Many workers have candy dishes on their desks. Get rid of yours immediately! Too often candy is mistaken for a quick energy source, a reward for accomplishing something, or simply something to eat when bored. Also, it is better to take the container away than leaving it empty. Many times, the sight of it will trigger a stimulus to get something sweet to eat.

98

Don't reach for food when you feel stressed. It is better to go for a short walk, squeeze a tennis ball, or simply take a few deep breaths to calm down.

99

Don't eat donuts, cookies, cakes or candy brought in by fellow workers. It's better to eat fruit as a snack if it is available. Even better yet; if you are in charge of bringing refreshments to a meeting, make sure to get fruit and other low calorie snacks. It will be a great change of pace in addition to helping you and others remain on your diets.

100

If a mobile lunch wagon serves your office or work place, don't automatically get up when it arrives blowing its whistle. (Remember the story about Pavlov's dogs salivating at the ringing of a bell?) The real purpose of that whistle is make you hungry and start you thinking about eating. Instead, when the whistle blows, go for a walk, do an errand, or make a telephone call. Try to associate the whistle with something other than food.

Final Tip ...

101

When dieting, always keep your mind focused on achieving your goal. One final way to do this is to think up your own personal ways to stay on your diet. If you've come across a good tip, we would like to hear from you. We will be happy to make you famous by giving you credit in our next edition. However, we do reserve the right to edit your tips and they become the property of the publisher. Please send your tips to: *Baker Publishing-Diet Tips, Post Office Box 8341 Mission Hills, CA 91346.*

Do a Friend a Favor

Pass a copy of this book along to a friend or family member, especially to someone who has been unsuccessful in losing weight and keeping it off. If you have trouble finding it at your local book store, additional copies can be ordered directly from the publisher. Send $4.95 plus $1.50 shipping to:

Baker Publishing
P.O. Box 8341
Mission Hills, CA 91346

Please include sales tax where applicable. Discounts are also available for multiple copy purchases.